Journey With God Through Suffering

Introduction

The goal of this handbook
is to help you and your group
lean on our Stronghold
as you journey with Him
through your crisis.

JOURNEY WITH GOD THROUGH SUFFERING
published by Stronghold Press, Dallas, Texas 75238.

© 2014 by Joe Fornear
ISBN 978-0-9840113-5-3
Cover and book design by Rebecca Horn, rhorngraphics

Unless otherwise indicated, Bible quotations are taken from The New American Standard Bible®, © 1995 by The Lockman Foundation. Used by permission. (www.Lockman.org).

Printed in the United States of America.

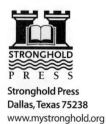

STRONGHOLD
PRESS

Stronghold Press
Dallas, Texas 75238
www.mystronghold.org

Table of Contents

Sovereignty

Embrace God's total control over all things.

KEY VERSES

Then Job arose and tore his robe and shaved his head,
and he fell to the ground and worshiped.
He said, "Naked I came from my mother's womb,
and naked I shall return there.
The LORD gave and the LORD has taken away.
Blessed be the name of the LORD."
Through all this Job did not sin nor did he blame God.
Job 1:20-22

Food for Thought

Do you think God causes pain in our lives?

_____

_____

_____

_____

_____

_____

_____

Purpose: The Lord is in control and we are not. He *allows* painful experiences and uses them to further His causes which are ultimately for our good and the good of others. So we need to cast all of our anxieties and fears upon Him. Then He will guard our hearts with His supernatural peace. (Philippians 4:6-7)

Travel Companion: John the Baptist

> *Now when John, while imprisoned, heard of the works of Christ, he sent word by his disciples and said to Him, "Are You the Expected One, or shall we look for someone else?"*
> *Jesus answered and said to them, "Go and report to John what you hear and see: the blind receive sight and the lame walk, the lepers are cleansed and the deaf hear, the dead are raised up, and the poor have the gospel preached to them. And blessed is he who does not take offense at Me."* Matthew 11:2-6

Jesus said John was the greatest man who had ever been born, but John could not understand why Jesus allowed him to remain in prison. After all, Jesus had the power to release him! Jesus responded that John needed to embrace His plan and not "stumble" over Jesus' choice to keep him imprisoned.

Respond: Surrender to that which He sovereignly allows us to suffer in life.

My Response

_____

_____

_____

_____

_____

_____

_____

Discuss/Consider

1. Do you think it is wrong to struggle or question God about our circumstances?

_____

_____

_____

_____

_____

_____

_____

2. How do we know if we have crossed the line from honest struggling into complaining and murmuring against God?

_____

_____

_____

_____

_____

_____

3. Are there other verses or Bible stories that help you embrace the
   sovereignty of God in your life?

_____

_____

_____

_____

_____

_____

_____

Journal

_____

_____

_____

_____

_____

_____

_____

_____

_____

_____

_____

_____

_____

_____

_____

_____

_____

_____

_____

_____

_____

_____

_____

_____

Trust

Believe in His goodness even in the midst of suffering.

KEY VERSES

How precious also are Your thoughts to me, O God!
How vast is the sum of them!
If I should count them, they would outnumber the sand.
Psalm 139:17-18

Food for Thought

If God is good, why does He allow suffering in our lives?

_____

_____

_____

_____

_____

_____

Purpose: To cling to the goodness of God even when we don't understand. The Lord is constantly thinking about us with tremendous love and compassion. Even though we don't understand all of His ways, He proved His ultimate love toward us by sending Jesus to die on the cross for us while we were yet sinners (Romans 5:8).

Travel Companion: Asaph

> _Will the Lord reject forever? And will He never be favorable again? Has His lovingkindness ceased forever? Has His promise come to an end forever? Has God forgotten to be gracious, or has He in anger withdrawn His compassion? Selah._
>
> _Then I said, "It is my grief, that the right hand of the Most High has changed."_
>
> _I shall remember the deeds of the LORD; Surely I will remember Your wonders of old. I will meditate on all Your work and muse on Your deeds. Your way, O God, is holy; What god is great like our God? You are the God who works wonders; You have made known Your strength among the peoples._
> Psalm 77:7-14

Because of a series of trials, Asaph felt he had been abandoned by the Lord. He was very upset and could not sleep (Psalm 77:4). He felt even worse when he concluded that God had changed (Psalm 77:10). Asaph's spirits lifted when he began to recount God's history of pouring out goodness on him and His people.

Respond: Stand firm that the Lord is always good, and recount the many times that He has blessed us. Always be thankful to Him for His ultimate expression of love for us sinners in the cross of Jesus Christ.

My Response

_____

_____

_____

_____

_____

_____

Discuss/Consider

1. Why do you think we so strongly connect His love with being pain-free?

_____

_____

_____

_____

_____

_____

2. Do you think we can make our trials more difficult by doubting His goodness?

_____

_____

_____

_____

_____

_____

_____

3. How does the cross of Christ factor into your understanding of the goodness of God?

_____

_____

_____

_____

_____

_____

_____

Journal

Rest

**Depend on His work and not on ours
for this life and eternal life.**

KEY VERSE

*For the one who has entered His rest
has himself also rested from his works, as God did from His.*
Hebrews 4:10

Food for Thought

Why do you think spiritual rest can be elusive?

_____

_____

_____

_____

Purpose: True spiritual rest begins with an eternal rest. The Bible basically describes two ways to get to heaven. The first is through our good works, but this way to heaven requires complete perfection:

> For as many as are of the works of the Law are under a curse; for it is written, "Cursed is everyone who does not abide by all things written in the book of the law to perform them" Galatians 3:10

> Whoever keeps the whole law and yet stumbles in one point, he has become guilty of all. James 2:10

Note that even one sin causes us to break the entire law and thereby fall under God's curse. The second way to get to heaven is through faith in Jesus' work—His sacrifice on the cross for our sins.

> For the wages of sin is death, but the free gift of God is eternal life in Christ Jesus our Lord. Romans 6:23

Note that eternal life is given to us as a "free gift."

Travel Companion: The thief on the cross did not deserve heaven, but received this free gift on his last day on earth.

> One of the criminals who were hanged there was hurling abuse at Him, saying, "Are You not the Christ? Save Yourself and us!"

> But the other answered, and rebuking him said, "Do you not even fear God, since you are under the same sentence of condemnation? And we indeed are suffering justly, for we are receiving what we deserve for our deeds; but this man has done nothing wrong."

> And he was saying, "Jesus, remember me when You come in Your kingdom!"

> And He said to him, "Truly I say to you, today you shall be with Me in Paradise." Luke 23:39-43

Respond: Receive the free gift of eternal life. Pray and ask Him to give it to you – He promises He will.

> *Behold, I stand at the door and knock; if anyone hears My voice and opens the door, I will come in to him and will dine with him, and he with Me.* Revelation 3:20

If you have already received His free gift, now ask Jesus to teach you how to rest in Him **as a lifestyle:**

> *"Come to Me, all who are weary and heavy-laden, and I will give you rest. Take My yoke upon you and learn from Me, for I am gentle and humble in heart, and you will find rest for your souls. For My yoke is easy and My burden is light."* Matthew 11:28-30

My Response

_____

_____

_____

_____

_____

_____

Discuss/Consider

1. What makes you feel spiritually rested?

_____

_____

_____

_____

_____

_____

_____

_____

2. Why do you think we want to earn God's blessings in this life and the next?

_____

_____

_____

_____

_____

_____

_____

3. How do you cease working?

_____

_____

_____

_____

_____

_____

_____

_____

Journal

Openness

**Admit and turn away from harmful
attitudes and behaviors.**

KEY VERSE

*Search me, O God, and know my heart;
Try me and know my anxious thoughts; and see if there be any
hurtful way in me, and lead me in the everlasting way.*
Psalms 139:23

Food for Thought

Why does God want us to admit or confess our sins?

_____

_____

_____

_____

_____

_____

Purpose: God knows everything about us and wants us to be free of harmful attitudes and behaviors toward Him, ourselves and others. We must allow Him to search and show us what sins we should admit and avoid.

Travel Companion: John

> _If we say that we have no sin, we are deceiving ourselves and the truth is not in us. If we confess our sins, He is faithful and righteous to forgive us our sins and to cleanse us from all unrighteousness. If we say that we have not sinned, we make Him a liar and His word is not in us._
> _My little children, I am writing these things to you so that you may not sin. And if anyone sins, we have an Advocate with the Father, Jesus Christ the righteous; and He Himself is the propitiation for our sins; and not for ours only, but also for those of the whole world._ 1 John 1:8-10; 2:1-2

John leads us to be honest with God and admit our sins. After we confess, we can claim the forgiveness and cleansing of Jesus Christ, who represents us before God our Father. Jesus' sacrifice on the cross was great enough to cover and wipe away all of our sins!

Respond: Be honest with God and make a list of your hurtful attitudes and behaviors. Then receive His forgiveness to wash away all guilt or shame from those sins.

My Response

_____

_____

_____

_____

_____

_____

_____

_____

Discuss/Consider

1. Why do you think confession is good for the soul?

_____

_____

_____

_____

_____

_____

_____

2. How can shame cause us to avoid admitting our sins to God?

_____

_____

_____

_____

_____

3. After you confess a sin, do you ever struggle with "feeling" forgiven? Do you struggle to forgive yourself?

_____

_____

_____

_____

_____

_____

_____

_____

_____

Journal

_____

_____

_____

_____

_____

_____

_____

_____

_____

_____

_____

_____

_____

_____

_____

_____

_____

_____

_____

_____

_____

_____

_____

_____

New Life

Depend on Christ's life and power inside of us.

KEY VERSE

*I have been crucified with Christ; and it is no longer I who live,
but Christ lives in me; and the life which I now live in the flesh I live
by faith in the Son of God, who loved me and gave Himself up for me.*
Galatians 2:20

Food for Thought

Why do you think we grow so weary in a crisis?

_____

_____

_____

_____

_____

_____

_____

Purpose: To grasp that we can do nothing apart from Christ, but we can do all things through Him.

Travel Companions: The disciples were called "branches" which are dependent on the vine, Jesus, in order to bear fruit.

> _Abide in Me, and I in you. As the branch cannot bear fruit of itself unless it abides in the vine, so neither can you unless you abide in Me. I am the vine, you are the branches; he who abides in Me and I in him, he bears much fruit, for apart from Me you can do nothing._ John 15:4-5

We were never intended to live the Christian life on our own, let alone battle a life-threatening crisis. The Father gave us Jesus to show us how to live but also to produce His very life and goodness in and through us. Jesus is an indwelling treasure.

Respond: Draw "life" and strength from Jesus Christ and not from our own limited resources.

My Response

_____

_____

_____

_____

_____

_____

_____

_____

_____

_____

Discuss/Consider

1. Have you ever been prideful in your ability to fight your own battles?

_____

_____

_____

_____

_____

_____

_____

2. What causes you to live independently from the Lord?

_____

_____

_____

_____

_____

_____

3. How do we grow in reliance on the Lord?

_____

_____

_____

_____

_____

_____

_____

_____

Journal

_____

_____

_____

_____

_____

_____

_____

_____

_____

_____

_____

_____

_____

_____

_____

_____

_____

_____

_____

_____

_____

_____

_____

_____

_____

_____

Grace

Extend forgiveness just as we have been forgiven.

KEY VERSE

Forgiving each other, just as God in Christ also has forgiven you.
Ephesians 4:32

Food for Thought

Is there someone who has hurt you and caused you grief?

_____

_____

_____

_____

_____

_____

Purpose: Release all of our grudges to God. Anger can be a healthy response to hurtful behavior. Still, we should not hold on to anger, but forgive just as Christ forgives us. When we hold grudges, we make our pain greater than God's ability to heal. This is a trap that will eventually cause us greater harm than the original hurt.

Travel Companions: The two slaves

> For this reason the kingdom of heaven may be compared to a king who wished to settle accounts with his slaves. When he had begun to settle them, one who owed him ten thousand talents [$6 billion U.S.] was brought to him. But since he did not have the means to repay, his lord commanded him to be sold, along with his wife and children and all that he had, and repayment to be made. So the slave fell to the ground and prostrated himself before him, saying, "Have patience with me and I will repay you everything."

> And the lord of that slave felt compassion and released him and forgave him the debt. But that slave went out and found one of his fellow slaves who owed him a hundred denarii [$10,000 U.S.]; and he seized him and began to choke him, saying, "Pay back what you owe."

> So his fellow slave fell to the ground and began to plead with him, saying, "Have patience with me and I will repay you." But he was unwilling and went and threw him in prison until he should pay back what was owed. So when his fellow slaves saw what had happened, they were deeply grieved and came and reported to their lord all that had happened.

Then summoning him, his lord said to him, "You wicked slave,
I forgave you all that debt because you pleaded with me.
Should you not also have had mercy on your fellow slave, in
the same way that I had mercy on you?" Matthew 18:23-33

Respond: Acknowledge the incredible debt of sin we have toward
God and how much He has forgiven us. Then forgive those who have
hurt you. Also pray a blessing on those who have hurt you as Jesus
instructs us in Luke 6:28-27.

My Response

_____

_____

_____

_____

_____

_____

_____

Discuss/Consider

1. Do you believe you have hurt God more than you have been hurt by
   others?

_____

_____

_____

_____

_____

_____

_____

_____

2. Do you believe that you hurt yourself more when you hold a grudge?

_____

_____

_____

_____

_____

_____

_____

3. Is it hard for you to extend grace to people who don't understand or who judge you because of your trials?

_____

_____

_____

_____

_____

_____

_____

_____

Journal

_____
_____
_____
_____
_____
_____
_____
_____
_____
_____
_____
_____
_____
_____
_____
_____
_____
_____
_____
_____
_____
_____
_____

Hope

Develop an eternal perspective.

KEY VERSE

He will wipe away every tear from their eyes;
and there will no longer be any death;
there will no longer be any mourning, or crying, or pain;
the first things have passed away.
Revelation 21:4

Food for Thought

Does looking forward to the ecstasy of heaven help lighten your
struggles now?

Purpose: Redirect our focus from the pain of this life which is
temporary, to the eternal relief and sheer joy which we will experience
in heaven—forever.

Travel Companion: Paul

> *Therefore we do not lose heart, but though our outer man is
> decaying, yet our inner man is being renewed day by day. For
> momentary, light affliction is producing for us an eternal
> weight of glory far beyond all comparison, while we look not
> at the things which are seen, but at the things which are not
> seen; for the things which are seen are temporal, but the things
> which are not seen are eternal. For we know that if the earthly
> tent which is our house is torn down, we have a building from
> God, a house not made with hands, eternal in the heavens. For
> indeed in this house we groan, longing to be clothed with our
> dwelling from heaven.* 2 Corinthians 4:16-5:2

Paul experienced an almost overwhelming amount of suffering. He
was beaten, stoned, robbed and imprisoned (2 Corinthians 11:23-
29). Yet he maintained a liberating eternal perspective, choosing to
focus on the lasting glory of heaven rather than the temporary and
"light" suffering of this world.

Respond: Focus on the eternal relief and joy of heaven as we journey with God through our temporary pain and suffering.

My Response

_____

_____

_____

_____

_____

_____

Discuss/Consider

1. Do you ever struggle with self-pity because of your pain and suffering?

_____

_____

_____

_____

_____

_____

2. What will it be like for you to see the Lord in person?

_____

_____

_____

_____

_____

_____

3. What do you think heaven will be like?

_____

_____

_____

_____

_____

_____

_____

_____

_____

Journal

_____

_____

_____

_____

_____

_____

_____

_____

_____

_____

_____

_____

_____

_____

_____

_____

_____

_____

_____

_____

_____

_____

_____

_____

_____

_____

_____

_____

_____

Omnipotence

The Lord wants us to ask Him to move our mountains.

KEY VERSES

And Jesus answered saying to them, "Have faith in God.
Truly I say to you, whoever says to this mountain, 'Be taken up and
cast into the sea,' and does not doubt in his heart,
but believes that what he says is going to happen, it will be granted him.
Therefore I say to you, all things for which you pray and ask,
believe that you have received them, and they will be granted you."
Mark 11:22-24

Food for Thought

Does prayer really make a difference?

_____

_____

_____

_____

_____

_____

_____

_____

Purpose: We should pray in the manner Jesus taught—with faith. When all verses on prayer in the Bible are considered, He does not absolutely guarantee to answer in the way we prefer. Still, He clearly delights when we boldly ask!

Travel Companion: James

> *You do not have because you do not ask.* James 4:2

> *But he must ask in faith without any doubting, for the one who doubts is like the surf of the sea, driven and tossed by the wind. For that man ought not to expect that he will receive anything from the Lord, being a double-minded man, unstable in all his ways.* James 1:6-8

James believed in prayer—his nickname was "camel knees," because his knees were so calloused from kneeling. He followed Jesus' admonition to boldly pray with faith, and miracles were common in his life.

Respond: Pray boldly believing He hears and will answer and then trust Him with the results.

My Response

_____

_____

_____

_____

_____

_____

Discuss/Consider

1. Do you believe God has the last word in your healing or are you discouraged by statistics, appearances or a doctor's prognosis?

_____

_____

_____

_____

_____

_____

2. Do you hesitate to ask God for healing because you are concerned about developing false hope?

_____

_____

_____

_____

_____

_____

3. Do you believe God still performs miracles today?

_____

_____

_____

_____

_____

_____

_____

_____

Journal

Laughter

Find joy in the midst of suffering.

KEY VERSES

Consider it all joy, my brethren, when you encounter various trials,
knowing that the testing of your faith produces endurance.
And let endurance have its perfect result,
so that you may be perfect and complete, lacking in nothing.
James 1:2-4

Food for Thought

Do you think it is possible to have joy in the midst of pain and hardship?

_____

_____

_____

_____

_____

_____

Purpose: Joy and laughter give hope by shifting our focus off us and our circumstances to God's promises of ultimate joy.

Travel Companion: Solomon

> *A joyful heart is good medicine, but a broken spirit dries up the bones.* Proverbs 17:22

Respond: Focus on being grateful and finding humor and joy in every circumstance. His supernatural joy is a gift and a fruit of His Holy Spirit within us. He will sustain us in hard times.

My Response

_____

_____

_____

_____

_____

_____

_____

Discuss/Consider

1. Do you find it insensitive that the Lord asks us to find joy in the midst
   of suffering?

_____

_____

_____

_____

_____

_____

2. How did joy motivate Jesus to endure suffering (Hebrews 12:2)?

_____

_____

_____

_____

_____

_____

_____

3. What have you done to find laughter in the midst of hard times?

_____

_____

_____

_____

_____

_____

_____

Journal

Display

Allow the life of the indwelling Christ to shine out to others.

KEY VERSES

*For God, who said, "Light shall shine out of darkness," is the
One who has shone in our hearts to give the Light of the knowledge
of the glory of God in the face of Christ. But we have this
treasure in earthen vessels, so that the surpassing greatness of the
power will be of God and not from ourselves; we are afflicted
in every way, but not crushed; perplexed, but not despairing; persecuted,
but not forsaken; struck down, but not destroyed; always
carrying about in the body the dying of Jesus, so that the life of Jesus
also may be manifested in our body. For we who live are
constantly being delivered over to death for Jesus' sake, so that the
life of Jesus also may be manifested in our mortal flesh.*
2 Corinthians 4:6-11

Food for Thought

Is it possible to glorify God even while we are suffering greatly?

_____

_____

_____

_____

_____

_____

_____

Purpose: Ultimately we exist to shine the life of Christ to others, not to live in comfort. This happens best through brokenness.

Travel Companion: Stephen

> *Now when they heard this, they were cut to the quick, and they began gnashing their teeth at him. But being full of the Holy Spirit, he gazed intently into heaven and saw the glory of God, and Jesus standing at the right hand of God; and he said, 'Behold, I see the heavens opened up and the Son of Man standing at the right hand of God."*
>
> *But they cried out with a loud voice, and covered their ears and rushed at him with one impulse. When they had driven him out of the city, they began stoning him; Acts 7:54-58*

Even while being stoned, Stephen focused on Jesus in heaven. He was glowing with the fullness of the Holy Spirit. He even prayed for their forgiveness, "Lord, do not hold this sin against them!" (Acts 7:60). People saw the Lord's light in Stephen and people can see the light of the Lord in us—especially during difficult times.

Respond: Focus on Christ to reflect His glory, even in the most difficult times.

My Response

_____

_____

_____

_____

_____

_____

_____

Discuss/Consider

1. What do you believe is your ultimate purpose in this life?

_____

_____

_____

_____

_____

_____

_____

2. Are you willing to suffer in order for God's light to shine to more people?

_____

_____

_____

_____

_____

_____

3. Will you see people in heaven who are there because you shared your
   faith in the Lord Jesus?

_____

_____

_____

_____

_____

_____

_____

_____

Journal